Natural **Organic Sunscreen**
15 Best Homemade Non-Toxic Sunscreen Recipes And 15 After-Sun Moisturizers

Table of content

Introduction

Summer is for lounging around by the pool, hitting the beach and going on holidays and let's be honest, for most of us the sun plays an important part in this. Everyone loves a sun tan which is a badge of pride that we have been somewhere warm and exotic and to many it is much more desirable. Women everywhere flock to the beach or even opt for synthetic spray tans or sun beds in the hopes of getting the illusive bronze look.

But what happens when you go too far? You get burnt. Many people don't realise that the sun can be just as damaging in the winter as it can in the summer and you need to protect your skin. Protecting your skin does not always mean you won't get a sun tan, but you must do it in the right way. Chapter 2 discussed what happens with regular unprotected exposure and the serious health implications.

Another common misconception is that you only need to apply sunscreen once and it will protect you. This is not true and is especially false for children who are generally in and out of the water or running around and rubbing off the protective layer. Kids are more susceptible to the negative impacts of the sun with as little as 2 hours unprotected midday sun can be life threatening if you do not properly protect them.

That being said, with the recipes in this eBook and the knowledge that you gain, there is no reason why you and your family can't enjoy summer the right way while being completely and naturally protected as possible.

Chapter 1 – The Importance of Skin Care

The sun is a daily part of our lives, we go outside all the time and there is usually little need for applying sunscreen every day (unless you spend long hours in the sun specifically). Many people believe that because of the daily exposure to the sun, the body builds up a tolerance and therefore does not need special protection and this is partly true. While generally you acclimatize to the level of natural exposure in your country (for example, those in Australia have a higher tolerance to the sun and are less likely to get burned due to their constant exposure compared to elsewhere such as England) which means you are at a lower risk to get burned, that does not reduce the risk that sun damage can cause.

UV radiation is what causes most forms of skin cancer including melanoma which is the most serious and difficult to treat (see below). Those who are in sunny climates whether the climate is warm or not can put you at extra risk of skin damaged caused by the UV exposure. For example, many skiers have to apply vast amounts of sunscreen to avoid getting burnt even in the extremely cold temperatures because the UV is amplified and is incredibly direct in those areas (perfect for skiing, not for the skin.)

Sun and UV exposure affects everyone and that is why you should always apply sunscreen if you are going to be in the sun for a prolonged amount of time, regardless of the weather. Many people underestimate the effect that continuous and unrestricted UV radiation has on the body and can cause many health issues such as;

Premature Skin Aging – Repetitive exposure to UV radiation (including from sunbeds) causes the skin to lose its elasticity and therefore it starts to sag, specifically in the face. In addition to this, it can cause the skin to have a "leather" feel after hardening due to prolonged sun damage. Those who are frequently out in the sun may actually start to appear older because the collagen in the skin starts to break down and does not rejuvenate as easily causing more rapid aging. In addition, the sagging tends to lead to bags and wrinkles, specifically under the eyes and in the neck area which can give a more tired appearance.

Tumors – Although many tumors as a result of UV radiation are actually benign, this can still cause health implications and rapid growth of skin cells that are abnormal. While this can also lead to cancer, benign tumors that grow in the wrong areas can cause thyroid issues, affect body functions and even mood swings. Benign tumors are usually also removed to prevent further growth and this would require surgery that could otherwise have been avoided.

Longer healing time – Skin that has been exposed to vast amounts of UV radiation has a damaged immune function response which means that it struggles to repair itself quickly. This can cause higher risks for surgery patients or those with other medical conditions and it can create problems for something as simple as a cut that is unable to heal as quickly. In addition, the skin is the first line of defense for viruses and bacteria which is compromised with repeated, unprotected exposure and will leave you more open to colds and infections if not properly protected.

Pigment Discoloration – In some cases, UV radiation can cause what is called mottled pigmentation which results in the skin losing some of the melanin and not producing anymore which means that parts of the skin become a lot lighter than other areas which gives a "patchy" skin tone. While this is not threatening to your health, the areas with the lack of melanin that are lighter are more prone to burning in the sun and can develop other skin issues such as dry flakey skin or eczema.

Skin Cancer – This is the big one that many know about and due to the lowered immune system and the promotion of abnormal cell growth, UV radiation is the leading cause of skin cancer. 2 out of 3 types of skin cancer are less serious and can be easily treated however melanoma is the most serious. It is responsible for over 70% of skin cancer related deaths because it is the type that is able to spread to other body organs quickly and is difficult to regulate. Children that are sun burned are at a higher risk of developing melanoma in their adult lives due to damaging the growing cells and immune system from a young age. Those with lighter skin or red or blonde hair are also at a higher risk due to less melanin pigment naturally occurring in their skin and those with darker skin and hair have less risk.

Direct sunlight without protection can also cause an array of other problems from sun stroke to dehydration which can all be severely taxing on the body and in some cases even fatal (especially in children). Sun burn is also a high risk, especially if you are changing climates and are not used to the level of sun exposure that you will be receiving. Getting sun burn can send your body into shock in the same way you would if you were exposed to a flame and can not only be incredibly painful but can cause a range of health implications as well. If you have experienced sun burn, chapters 17-31 should contain the recipes to soothe and rejuvenate the skin and chapters 2-16 should be able to prevent this from happening in the future.

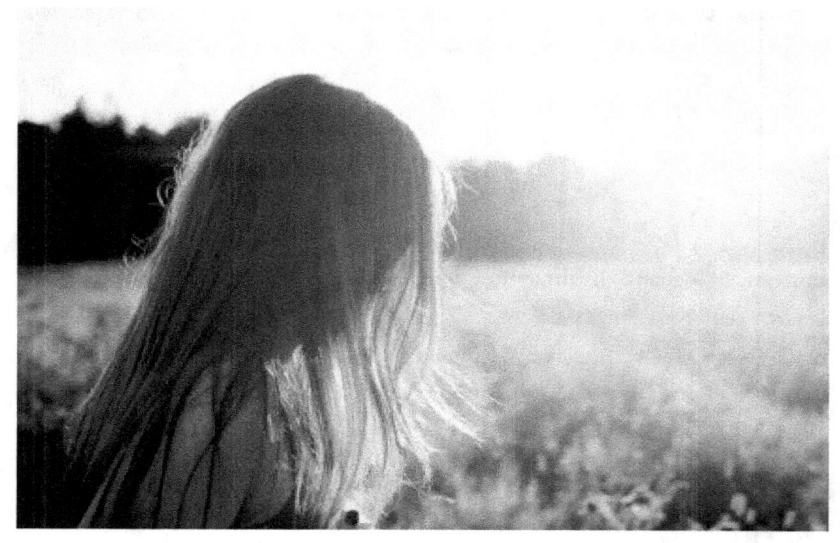

Chapter 2 – Jojoba Oil Sun cream

<u>You will need</u>

- 1 ounce of Coconut Oil

- Zinc Oxide Powder (follow instructions for quantities depending on brand)

- 0.1 Ounce of Jojoba Oil

- 1 Ounce of Shea Butter

- 1 ½ Tablespoons Eucalyptus Essential Oil

- 0.1 Ounce Vitamin E Oil

<u>Method</u>

1. Add the coconut oil, Shea butter and jojoba oil to a double boiler and melt gently together but do not allow to bubble.

2. Allow it to cool and add the vitamin E oil, essential oil and zinc powder to the mixture and stir together until all ingredients are combined.

3. Keep in the fridge in a darkened jar.

<u>Notes</u>:

Make sure to use a mask or protective equipment to avoid inhaling the zinc oxide powder.

<u>To Use</u>:

Apply to skin that is exposed to sunlight and make sure to use liberally and reapply frequently to maintain protection.

Chapter 3 - Almond Sunscreen

You will need

* 1 ounce of Coconut Oil

* Zinc Oxide Powder (follow instructions for quantities depending on brand)

* 0.1 Ounce of Sunflower Oil

* 0.8 Ounces of Almond Butter

* 0.1 Ounce Vitamin E Oil

Method

1. Add the coconut oil, almond butter and sunflower oil to a double boiler and melt gently together but do not allow to bubble.

2. Allow it to cool and add the vitamin E oil and zinc powder to the mixture and stir together until all ingredients are combined

3. Keep in the fridge in a darkened jar.

Notes:

* Make sure to use a mask or protective equipment to avoid inhaling the zinc oxide powder.

* Should Last approximately 6 months

To Use:

Apply to skin that is exposed to sunlight and make sure to use liberally and reapply frequently to maintain protection.

Chapter 4 – Lavender Sunscreen

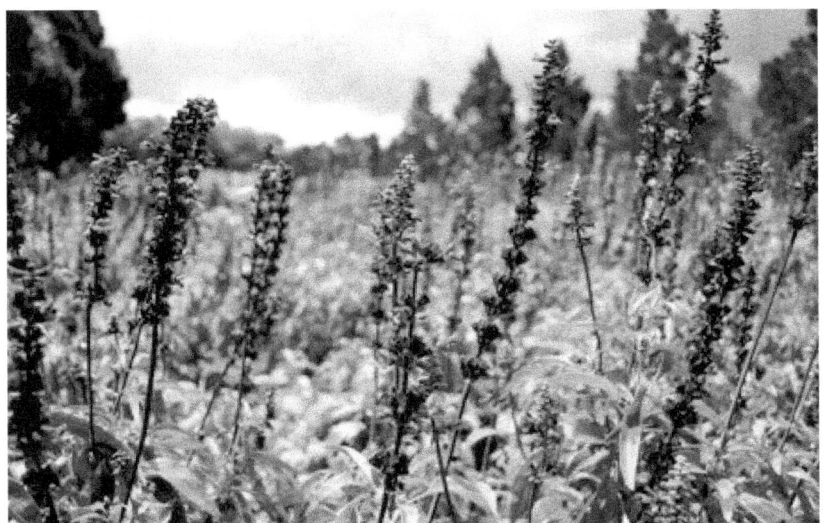

Photo Source: Free Stock Photo

<u>You will need</u>

½ Cup of Olive Oil

1/8 Cup Lavender Flower

¼ Cup of Beeswax

¼ Cup of Coconut Oil

2 Tablespoons Zinc Oxide Powder

1 Teaspoon Vitamin E Oil

1 ½ Tablespoons Lavender Essential Oil

Method

1. Infuse the olive oil and the lavender heads together and then strain when done to remove the excess plant material.

2. Add all of the ingredients (except the zinc oxide) into a double boiler and gently melt them together while stirring occasionally.

3. Remove from the heat and now add the zinc oxide powder

4. Stir and place in a jar or tin to store.

Notes:

- Use within 6 months

- Do not keep in direct sunlight

- Make sure to use a mask or protective equipment to avoid inhaling the zinc oxide powder.

Chapter 5 – Peppermint Oil Sun Cream

<u>You will need</u>

- ¼ Cup of Almond Oil

- ¼ Cup of Beeswax

- 2 Tbsp. Shea Butter

- 1 Tsp Peppermint Essential Oil

- 1 Tsp Carrot Seed Oil

- 2 Tablespoons Zinc Oxide Powder

- 1 Tsp Vitamin E Oil

- ¼ Cup of Coconut Oil

<u>Method</u>

1. Add the Shea butter, beeswax and almond oil to a double boiler and stir until completely melted.

2. Add the essential oil, carrot seed oil, vitamin E and coconut oil and stir further until completely mixed.

3. Remove from the heat and add the zinc oxide powder.

4. Transfer to darkened storage glass jars or tins

<u>Notes</u>:

- Use within 6 months

- Do not store in direct sunlight

- Refrigerate

- Make sure to use a mask or protective equipment to avoid inhaling the zinc oxide powder.

Chapter 6 – Soothing Eucalyptus Sunscreen

<u>You will need</u>

- 1 Teaspoon of Red Raspberry Seed Oil

- 2 Teaspoons Eucalyptus Oil

- ½ Cup Olive Oil

- ¼ Cup Shea Butter

- 2 Tablespoons Zinc Oxide Powder

- 1 Teaspoon Vitamin E Oil

- 1 Teaspoon Peppermint Essential Oil

- 2 Tablespoons Beeswax

<u>Method</u>

1. Add the Shea butter and beeswax to a double boiler and melt. (stir occasionally)

2. Add the oils and stir again until completely mixed

3. Remove from the heat and then add the zinc oxide powder. Stir until completely mixed.

4. Transfer to darkened storage containers.

<u>Notes</u>:

- Do not use in direct sunlight

- Make sure to use a mask or protective equipment to avoid inhaling the zinc oxide powder.

Photo Source: Free Stock Image

Chapter 7 – Pomegranate Shea Sun Cream

You will need

- 2 Tablespoons Shea Butter

- 1 Tablespoon Pomegranate Oil

- 2 Teaspoons Lavender Essential Oil

- 2 Tablespoons Zinc Oxide powder

- ¾ Cup Coconut Oil

Method

1. Using a double boiler, melt together the Shea butter and coconut oil and stir occasionally.

2. Stir in the pomegranate and lavender oil until completely mixed in.

3. Remove from the heat and add the zinc oxide powder making sure to carefully stir it in.

Notes:

- Store in a glass jar in the fridge

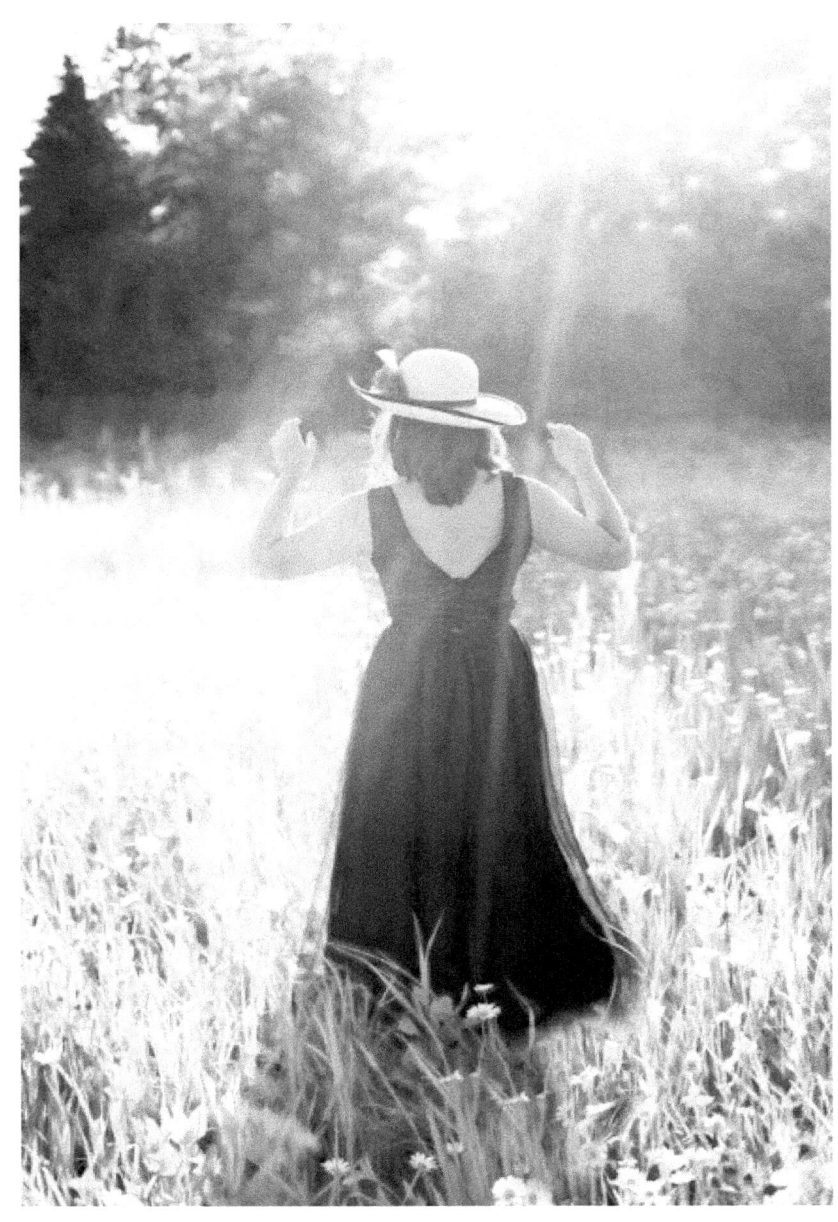

- Make sure to use a mask or protective equipment to avoid inhaling the zinc oxide powder.

Chapter 8– Natural Tinted Avocado Oil Sunscreen

<u>You will need</u>

- ¾ Cup Avocado Oil

- 3 Tbsp. Beeswax

- ¾ Cup Rose Water

- 2 Teaspoons Cocoa Powder (natural tinting agent)

- 3 Tablespoons Zinc Oxide Powder

- 1 Teaspoon Rose Essential Oil (optional)

<u>Method</u>

1. Add the avocado oil, beeswax and rose water to a double boiler and use a medium heat to mix all of the ingredients together, making sure to stir thoroughly.

2. Add the essential oil (if using) and mix together completely.

3. Remove from the heat and add the cocoa powder and zinc oxide powder to the mixture and stir until completely combined.

4. Allow to cool and store in the fridge.

<u>Notes</u>

Always use protective clothing or equipment when handling zinc oxide powder and do not inhale.

Chapter 9 – Coconut Grapeseed Oil Sunscreen

<u>You will need</u>

* 7 Ounces Grapeseed Oil

* 1 Ounce Coconut Oil

* 1.5 Ounces Beeswax

* 1 Teaspoon Coconut Essential Oil

* 2 Tablespoons Micronized Titanium Dioxide

<u>Method</u>

1. Using a double boiler, melt the beeswax, coconut oil and grapeseed oil together and mix until completely combined.

2. Add the essential oil and stir in thoroughly.

3. Remove the mixture from the heat and add the titanium dioxide, make sure to thoroughly stir in and mix all of the particles.

4. Allow to cool and store in a darkened glass jar.

<u>Notes</u>

* Make sure not to breathe in the titanium dioxide and wear protective clothing when handling as it can be an irritant.

Chapter 10– Beeswax Sunscreen with Vitamin E

You will need

- ½ Cup Coconut Oil

- 1/8 Cup Beeswax

- 1/8 Cup Shea Butter

- 1/3 Cup Jojoba Oil

- 3 Tablespoons Zinc Oxide Powder

- ½ Teaspoon Vitamin E Oil

Method

1, Using a double boiler, heat the coconut oil, beeswax and Shea butter together making sure that you mix occasionally.

2. Once combined, add the jojoba oil and vitamin E oil to the mixture and mix together completely.

3. Remove the mixture from the heat and stir in the zinc oxide powder thoroughly.

4. Allow to cool and store in a cool place.

Notes

- Make sure to use a mask or protective equipment to avoid inhaling the zinc oxide powder.

- Ensure to re-apply liberally to maintain protection

Chapter 11 – Coconut & Apricot Sunscreen

<u>You will need</u>

- ½ Cup Apricot Oil

- 1/8 Cup Beeswax

- 1/3 Cup Almond Oil

- 1/8 Cup Shea Butter

- 4 Tablespoons Zinc Oxide Powder

- 2 Teaspoons Coconut Oil

- ½ Teaspoon Coconut Essential Oil (optional)

<u>Method</u>

1. Place all of the ingredients (apart from the zinc oxide powder) into a bowl and heat using a double boiler.

2. Stir frequently until all of the ingredients are combined

3. Remove from the heat and carefully mix in the zinc oxide powder.

<u>Notes</u>

- Store in the refrigerator for no more than 6 months

- Make sure to use a mask or protective equipment to avoid inhaling the zinc oxide powder.

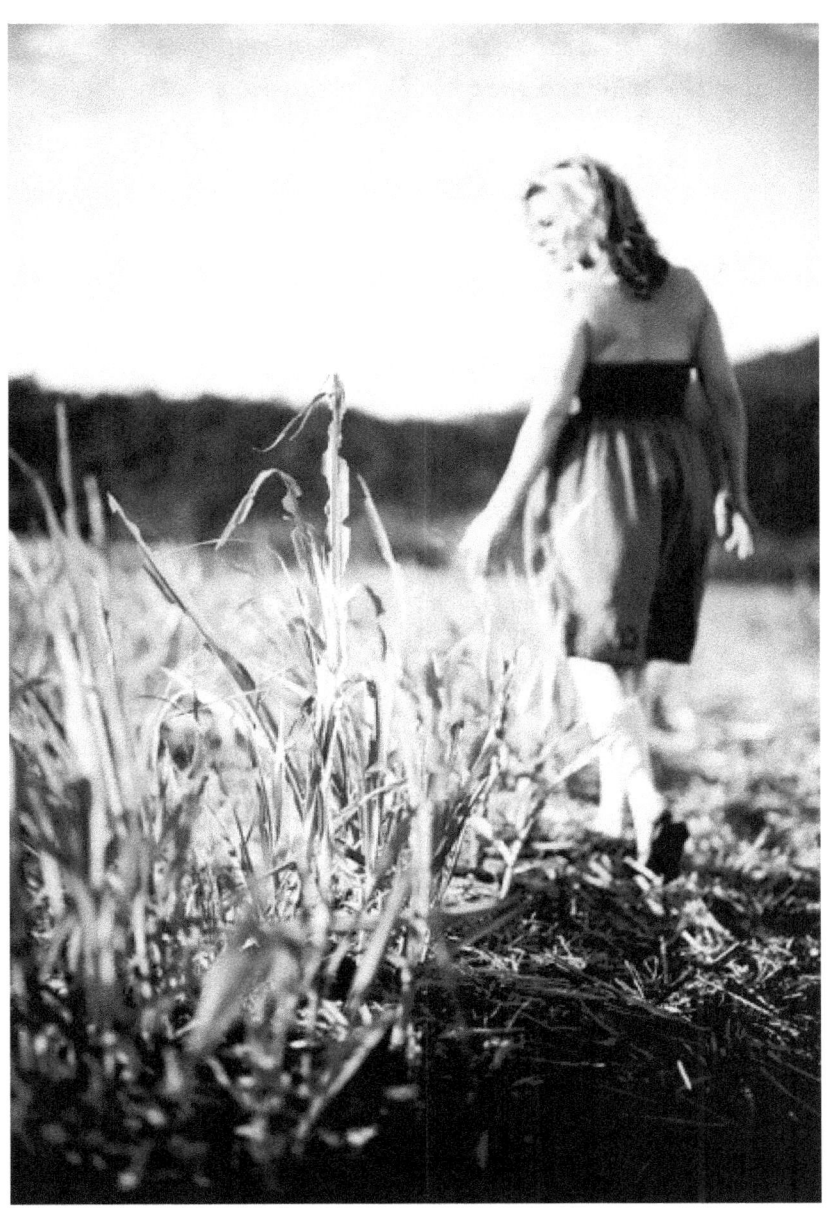

Chapter 12 – Mint and Shea Butter Sun Cream

<u>You will need</u>

- 1 Ounce Coconut Oil

- 1 Ounce of Olive Oil

- 1 Teaspoon Mint Leaves

- 1 Ounce Zinc Oxide Powder

- 2 Ounces Shea Butter

- ½ Teaspoon Peppermint Essential Oil

<u>Method</u>

1. Infuse the olive oil with the mint leaves by mixing them and leaving them overnight.

2. Strain the mixture and discard the plant material.

3. Add all of the ingredients to a double boiler (apart from the Zinc oxide) and mix together completely, making sure to stir frequently.

4. When completely combined, remove from the heat and gently stir in the zinc oxide powder.

5. Allow to cool and store in darkened jars.

<u>Notes</u>:

- Make sure to use a mask or protective equipment to avoid inhaling the zinc oxide powder.

Chapter 13 – Calendula Infused Sun Cream

<u>You will need</u>

- ½ Cup Olive Oil
- 4 Tablespoons Calendula
- ¼ Cup Coconut Oil
- 1/8 Cup Beeswax
- ½ Cup Shea Butter
- 1 Tsp Vitamin E Oil
- 2 Teaspoons Zinc Oxide Powder

<u>Method</u>

1. Infuse the calendula and olive oil by steeping the flowers overnight. In the morning remove the plant material.

2. Add the infused oil, beeswax, Shea butter and coconut oil to a double boiler and soften, mixing frequently.

3. Add the vitamin E oil and stir until mixed thoroughly.

4. Remove from the heat and carefully add the zinc oxide powder.

5. Transfer to storage jars and allow to completely cool before using.

<u>Notes</u>:

- Store for less than 6 months in the fridge

- Apply frequently and liberally

- Make sure to use a mask or protective equipment to avoid inhaling the zinc oxide powder.

Chapter 14– Sun Cream with Aloe Vera

You will need

- 1/8 Cup Avocado Oil

- 1/8 Cup Beeswax

- ¼ Cup Shea Butter

- ½ Cup Aloe Vera (the best format is gel)

- 2 Teaspoons Zinc Oxide Powder

- ½ Cup Coconut Oil

- 2 Teaspoons Lavender Essential Oil

Method

1. Add all of the ingredients to a double boiler except the zinc oxide powder and soften.

2. Stir frequently until all of the ingredients are completely mixed together.

3. Remove from the heat and stir in the zinc oxide powder until mixed in

4. Allow to cool and add to darkened glass jars

Notes:

- Store in the fridge

- Make sure to use a mask or protective equipment to avoid inhaling the zinc oxide powder.

Chapter 15 – Cocoa Butter Sunscreen

You will need

- ¼ Cup Cocoa Butter

- ¼ Cup Coconut Oil

- 1 ½ Teaspoons Red Raspberry Seed Oil

- 1/8 Cup Beeswax

- 1 Teaspoon Cocoa Powder (Optional for tint)

- 2 Teaspoons Zinc Oxide Powder

Method

1. Add the cocoa butter, beeswax and coconut oil to a double boiler and melt together thoroughly.

2. Stirring frequently add the raspberry seed oil and cocoa powder (if using) and stir until all the ingredients are thoroughly combined.

3. Take the mixture off of the heat and stir in the zinc oxide powder until thoroughly mixed and transfer to the storage tin or jar and allow to cool.

Notes:

- Store in a cool place

- Make sure to use a mask or protective equipment to avoid inhaling the zinc oxide powder.

Chapter 16 – Sesame and Coconut Sunscreen

<u>You will need</u>

- 1/8 Cup Olive Oil

- 1/8 Cup Neem Oil

- ¼ Cup Coconut Oil

- ¼ Cup Sesame Oil

- ¼ Cup Shea Butter

- 2 Teaspoons Zinc Oxide Powder

- 1 Teaspoon Vitamin E Oil

- 1 Teaspoon Eucalyptus Oil

- ¼ Cup Beeswax

<u>Method</u>

1. Add all of the ingredients to a double boiler except the zinc oxide powder and melt together making sure to stir frequently.

2. Once all of the ingredients are combined, remove the mixture from the heat and carefully add the zinc oxide power.

3. Stir it in completely and transfer to a darkened glass jar and store in the fridge.

<u>Notes</u>:

- Apply liberally and reapply every couple of hours

- Make sure to use a mask or protective equipment to avoid inhaling the zinc oxide powder.

After-Sun Recipes

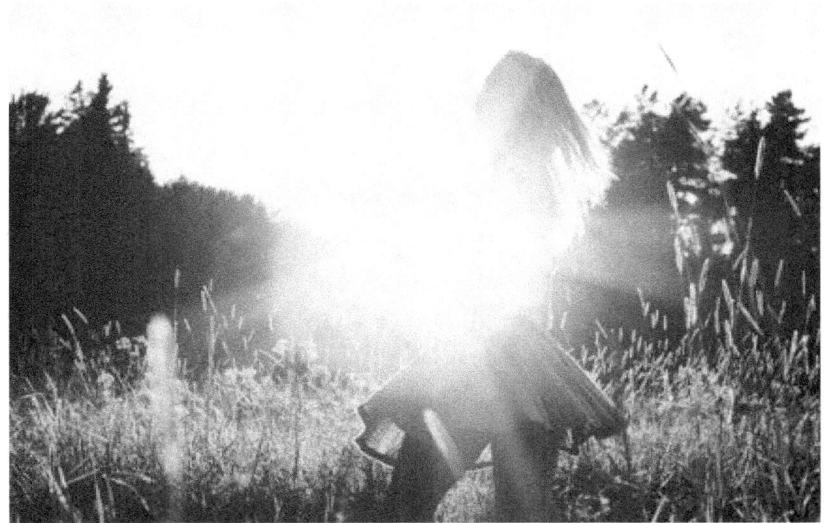

Photo Source: Free Stock Image

Chapter 17 – Aloe & Olive Oil After-Sun Lotion

<u>You will need</u>

- 1 Tbsp. Olive Oil

- 1 Tbsp. Shea butter

- 2 Tbsp. Coconut Oil

- 3 ½ Tbsp. Aloe Vera Gel

- 1 Teaspoon Eucalyptus Essential Oil

<u>Method</u>

1. Mix all of the ingredients in a bowl and stir until completely blended.

2. If the coconut oil or Shae butter is too hard you may need to warm it gently before mixing.

<u>Notes</u>

- Store in a darkened tin or glass jar

- Apply liberally

Chapter 18 – Cooling Peppermint After-sun Spray

<u>You will need</u>

- 4 Tablespoons Aloe Vera Gel

- Distilled Water

- 1 Tablespoon Apple Cider Vinegar (Raw)

- 6 Tablespoons Peppermint Hydrosol

- 2 Teaspoons Peppermint Essential Oil

- 8 Ounce Spray Bottle

- Optional: ½ Tablespoon Colloidal Silver (for extreme sunburn this helps to reduce infection)

<u>Method</u>

1. Mix all of the ingredients together and pour in the spray bottle.

2. Fill it up the rest of the way with the distilled water

3. Shake well and place in the fridge

<u>Notes</u>:

- Keep refrigerated

- Spray regularly to the affected area

- Avoid the eyes

- Do not use on children under 6

Chapter 19– Lavender Mist After-Sun Spray

<u>You will need</u>

- Distilled or purified water

- 1 Tablespoon Apple Cider Vinegar (Raw)

- 2 Teaspoons Lavender Oil

- 4 Tablespoons Aloe Vera Gel

- ½ Tablespoon Colloidal Silver

- ½ Tablespoon Vegetable Glycerin

- 8 Ounce Spray Bottle

<u>Method</u>

1. Add all of the ingredients to a bowl and mix thoroughly.

2. Pour into the spray bottle and top up with distilled or purified water.

3. Shake the bottle and refrigerate before using.

<u>Notes</u>:

- Do not spray in the eyes

- Keep refrigerated between uses

Chapter 20– Shea After-Sun Body Lotion

<u>You will need</u>

- 5 Tablespoons Shea Butter

- 1 Tablespoon Almond butter

- 3 Tablespoons Olive Oil

- 2 Tablespoons Aloe Vera Gel

- 1 Tablespoons Coconut Oil

<u>Method</u>

1. Add all of the ingredients into a bowl and stir until completely mixed.

2. Add to a storage container and leave in the fridge to allow it to gain some solidity

<u>Notes</u>

- You can use this recipe by itself or you can add it to your own organic body lotion and give it an extra boost.

- Use within 3-6 months

Chapter 21– Lavender & Aloe After-sun Oil

<u>You will need</u>

- 1 Teaspoon Lavender Blossom

- 2 Tablespoons Aloe Vera Gel

- 1 Teaspoon Lavender Essential Oil

- 3 Tablespoons Olive Oil

- 1 Tsp Cocoa Butter

- 1 Tsp Shea Butter

- 2 Tablespoons Beeswax

- 1 Teaspoon Coconut Oil

<u>Method</u>

1. Infuse the lavender blossom into the olive oil by steeping the flower overnight.

2. Drain and discard the leftover flowers.

3. Add the ingredients (including the infused olive oil) to a double boiler (except the Aloe Vera gel) and melt together until mixed.

4. Stir frequently and remove from the heat

5. Add the Aloe Vera gel and stir together thoroughly

6. Transfer to a container and store in the fridge

<u>Notes:</u>

Apply liberally and as regularly as needed

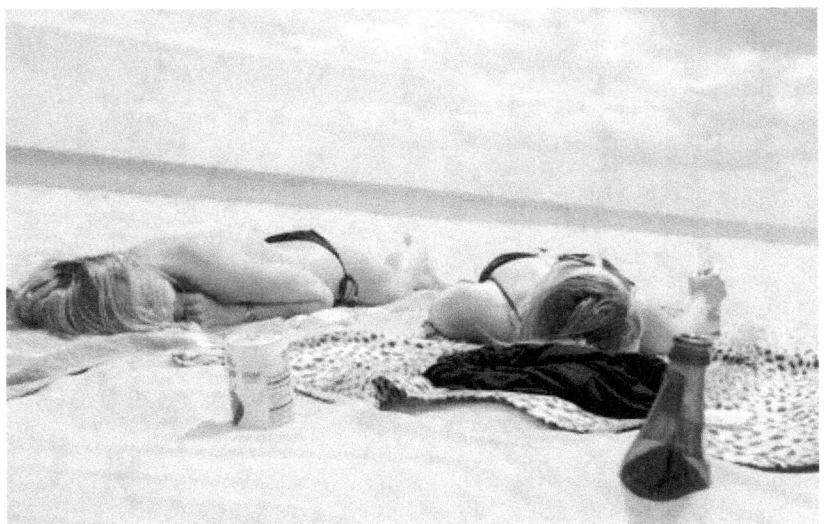

Photo Source: Free Stock Image

Chapter 22 – Calendula Butter After-Sun Oil

<u>You will need</u>

- 3 Tablespoons Olive Oil

- 1 Tablespoons Calendula Flowers

- 2 Tablespoons Cocoa Butter

- 2 Tablespoons Beeswax

- 2 Tablespoons Aloe Vera Gel

- 2 Teaspoons Eucalyptus Essential Oil

<u>Method</u>

1. Add the calendula flowers to the olive oil and vigorously stir for a few minutes.

2. Leave for an hour and then strain to remove the extra flowers

3. Add the butter and beeswax to a double boiler and heat until melted and mixed

4. Add the infused olive oil and essential oil to the mixture and stir completely

5. Remove from the heat and stir in the Aloe Vera gel

<u>Notes</u>:

- Store in the fridge in between uses

- Apply liberally to the affected area

Chapter 23 – Coconut & Eucalyptus After-Sun Lotion

<u>You will need</u>

- 4 Teaspoons Aloe Vera

- 4 Teaspoons Coconut Oil

- 1 Teaspoon Olive Oil

- 2 Teaspoons Shea Butter

- ½ Teaspoon Eucalyptus Essential Oil

<u>Method</u>

1. Add all of the ingredients into a bowl and beat together as you would with butter.

2. Combine all of the ingredients stir vigorously.

3. Place in a container and allow to set in the fridge overnight

<u>Notes</u>:

- Store in a cool, dry place

- Apply liberally

Chapter 24 – Olive Oil & Peppermint After-Sun Lotion

<u>You will need</u>

- 2 ½ Tablespoons Aloe Vera Gel

- 1 Tablespoon Almond Butter

- 1 Tablespoon Shea Butter

- 3 Tablespoons Olive Oil

- 1 Tablespoon Coconut Oil

- ½ Teaspoon Peppermint Essential Oil

<u>Method</u>

1. In a bowl, place all of the ingredients and beat together until smooth and creamy.

2. Transfer to a storage container and leave in a cool place. If you have a runnier texture then allow to set in the fridge overnight.

<u>Notes</u>:

- Apply topically whenever needed

Chapter 25 – Shea and Coconut After-sun Lotion

<u>You will need</u>

- 2 Tablespoons Shea Butter

- 3 Tablespoons Coconut Oil

- 2 ½ Tablespoons Aloe Vera

- 1 Teaspoon Lavender Essential Oil

- ½ Teaspoon Vitamin E Oil

- 1 Teaspoon Olive Oil

<u>Method</u>

1. Beat all of the ingredients together in a bowl and stir thoroughly until completely mixed.

2. Transfer to a storage container and leave in the fridge overnight to set

<u>Notes</u>

- Apply liberally every few hours on the affected area

Chapter 26 – Aloe & Witch Hazel After-Sun Spray

You will need

- 8 Tablespoons Fresh Aloe Pulp (from the plant)

- 5 Tablespoons Distilled Water

- 5 Tablespoons Witch Hazel

- ½ Teaspoon Eucalyptus Essential Oil

- 2 Tablespoons Vitamin E Oil

- 4 Ounce Spray bottle

Method

1. Combine the pulp, vitamin E and eucalyptus oil in a bowl and mix together thoroughly. Break apart any large clumps.

2. Pour the water and witch hazel into the mixture making sure to stir in completely.

3. Pour into the spray bottle and shake vigorously

Notes:

- Keep out of eyes

- Store in the fridge for extra cooling effect

- Will last 1-2 months

Photo Source: Free Stock Image

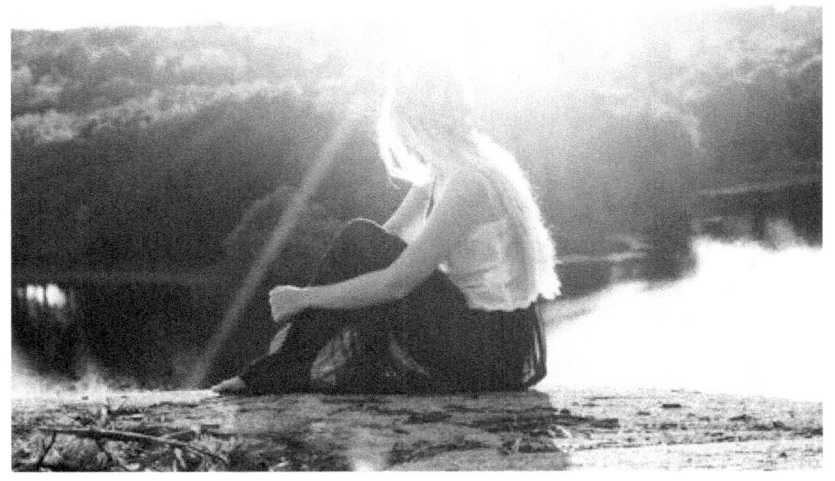

Chapter 27 – Chamomile After-Sun Lotion

<u>You will need</u>

- 2 Tablespoons St. John's Wort Oil

- 3 Tablespoons Olive Oil

- 2 Teaspoons Calendula Flowers

- 2 Tablespoons Chamomile Oil

- 1 Tablespoons Cocoa Butter

- 2 Tablespoons Beeswax

<u>Method</u>

1. Infuse the olive oil with the calendula flowers by stirring the two together and leaving them overnight.

2. Remove and discard the leftover plant material.

3. In a double boiler, melt together the cocoa butter, infused olive oil and beeswax, making sure to stir regularly until mixed together.

4. Add the St. John's Wort and chamomile oil and stir completely.

5. Allow to cool and transfer to a container and leave in the fridge

<u>Notes</u>:

- Apply liberally to affected area

- Store in the fridge and use within 2 months

Chapter 28 – Cocoa Butter & Rose After-Sun Lotion

<u>You will need</u>

- 2 Tablespoons Cocoa Butter

- 1 Tablespoon Beeswax

- 2 Tablespoons Aloe Vera Gel

- 2 Tablespoons Rose Water

- 1 Tablespoon Chamomile Oil

<u>Method</u>

1. Add all of the ingredients to a double boiler and gently heat until mixed together

2. Pour the mixture into a storage container and place in the fridge overnight to set before using.

<u>Notes</u>:

- Keep refrigerated

- Use within 1-2 months

Chapter 29 – Lavender & Witch Hazel After-Sun Spray

You will need

- 8 Tablespoons Aloe Vera Gel

- 1 ½ Teaspoons Lavender Essential Oil

- 2 Tablespoons Vitamin E Oil

- 4 Tablespoons Witch Hazel

- 6 Tablespoons Distilled or Purified Water

- 4 Ounce Spray Bottle

Method

1. Add the aloe gel, lavender and vitamin E oils to a bowl and stir together

2. Combine the witch hazel and stir into the mixture

3. Pour into the spray bottle and top up the rest with the distilled water

4. Shake vigorously and store in the fridge overnight before use.

Notes:

- Keep in the fridge for a cooling effect

- Keep out of eyes

- Use to soothe sunburnt skin

Chapter 30 – Simple 3 Ingredient After-sun Oil

<u>You will need</u>

- 2 Tablespoons Almond Oil

- ½ Teaspoon Eucalyptus Essential Oil

- 2 Tablespoons Almond Oil

- Spray Bottle

<u>Method</u>

1. Add all of the ingredients into the spray bottle and vigorously shake.

2. Keep in the fridge for an extra cooling effect

<u>Notes</u>

- Keep out of the eyes

- There is no need to wash this spray off, just allow it to soak into the skin naturally

Chapter 31 – Regeneration After-sun Butter

<u>You will need</u>

- 1 Tablespoon Shea Butter

- 1 Tablespoon Avocado Butter

- 2 Tablespoons Aloe Vera Pulp

- 1 Tablespoon Evening Primrose Oil

- 2 Teaspoons Eucalyptus Oil

- 1 Teaspoon Vitamin E Oil

<u>Method</u>

1. Add all of the ingredients into a bowl and beat together thoroughly. You may find you need to gently heat them to mix properly.

2. Once stirred and completely combined, transfer to a storage container and leave in the fridge overnight before the first use.

<u>Notes:</u>

- Store in the fridge

- Apply liberally and frequently to the affected area

Photo Source: Free Stock Image

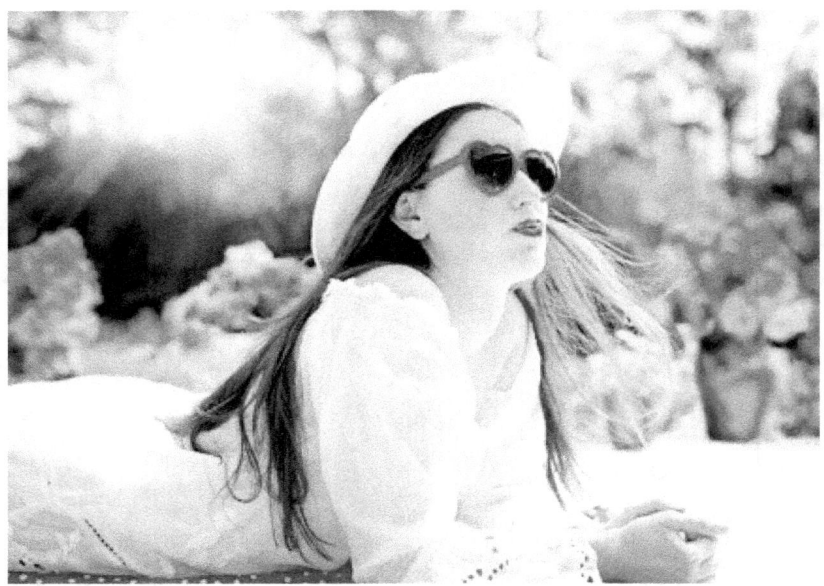

Conclusion

Hopefully this eBook has given you all the insight you need into the best ways to naturally protect yourself and your family from the sun. Using these recipes you can be safe in the knowledge that you can enjoy the sunshine and summer without any of the detrimental health risks. In addition to this you no longer have to be concerned about the chemicals that you exposing to yourself and family due to the commercial products on the market. You can also enjoy experimenting with these recipes to find the right texture, fragrance and protection that is right for you and you can easily adapt them for larger or smaller families. Finally, don't fall prey to the sun and enjoy it while being thoroughly protected.

Thanks for reading.

FREE Bonus Reminder

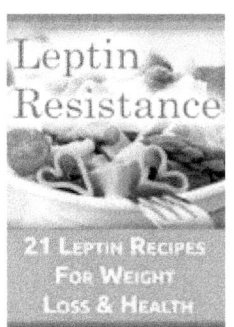

If you have not grabbed it yet, please go ahead and download your special bonus report *"Leptin Resistance. 21 Leptin Recipes For Weight Loss & Healthy Living"*.

Simply Click the Button Below

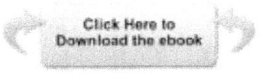

OR **Go to This Page**

http://easyweightlossway.com/free/

BONUS #2: More Free & Discounted Books

Do you want to receive more Free & Discounted Books?

We have a mailing list where we send out our new Books when they go free or with a discount on Kindle. Click on the link below to sign up for Free & Discount Book Promotions.

=> Sign Up for Free & Discount Book Promotions <=

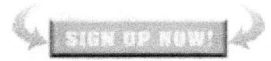

OR Go to this URL

http://zbit.ly/1WBb1Ek